UNDERSTANDING CHRONIC FATIGUE SYNDROME

Comprehensive Guide To Symptoms, Causes, Diagnosis, And Effective Management Strategies For Lasting Relief

DR. LINCOLN WAYLON

DISCLAIMER

This book contains information that should only be used for educational and informational reasons; it is not meant to be used as a source of medical or psychological advice. The author's studies, life experiences, and expertise in the area of health and wellness served as the foundation for the content. It should not, however, be used in place of expert counsel, a diagnosis, or medical care.

Any queries you may have about a physical or mental health issue should always be directed toward the advice of a licensed healthcare provider or mental health specialist. With regard to the efficacy or outcomes of the methods or suggestions included in this book, the author and publisher make no representations or warranties.

Any information or methods in this book are used entirely at the reader's own risk and discretion. The material provided here may be used or misused, and neither the author nor the publisher will be held responsible for any results, losses, or negative impacts.

Keep in mind that everyone has different demands and reactions to health and wellness routines. Any health and wellness plans you implement must be customized to your particular circumstances, and you should speak with experts to make sure the plans meet your needs.

TABLE OF CONTENTS

ABOUT THE BOOK

The book Understanding Chronic Fatigue Syndrome serves as a crucial resource for anyone grappling with the complexities of this often misunderstood condition. Chronic Fatigue Syndrome (CFS) is characterized by persistent, unexplained fatigue that profoundly impacts daily functioning. This book offers a comprehensive overview of CFS, delineating its key symptoms and diagnostic criteria, and distinguishing it from other fatigue disorders. By emphasizing the importance of accurate diagnosis, it highlights how critical it is for individuals to recognize the significant impact CFS can have on their daily lives.

A central focus of the book is on medical diagnosis and testing, offering a detailed examination of diagnostic criteria and common tests. It clarifies the role of primary care physicians and specialists in diagnosing CFS, providing guidance on interpreting test results and navigating the path to an accurate diagnosis.

This segment is particularly valuable for individuals seeking clarity on their condition and those advocating for appropriate medical attention.

Treatment and management of CFS are explored through various approaches, including medications, supplements, lifestyle modifications, and therapies such as cognitive-behavioral therapy (CBT).

The book also addresses managing coexisting conditions, offering a holistic approach to treatment that integrates both medical and lifestyle strategies. Self-care is underscored as an essential component, with practical advice on dietary recommendations, exercise, stress management, and sleep hygiene tailored to the needs of those with CFS.

Building a support network is another critical aspect covered, guiding readers in finding support groups, involving family and friends, and leveraging online communities. The book emphasizes the importance of advocacy and raising awareness, empowering readers to seek the support and resources they need.

Navigating the healthcare system is a complex journey, and this book provides invaluable insights into working with healthcare providers, understanding insurance coverage, and managing medical appointments. It encourages self-advocacy and offers strategies for effectively navigating medical settings.

For those balancing work and education with CFS, the book addresses legal rights, accommodations, and strategies for productivity and energy management. It provides practical advice for managing CFS in the workplace and educational settings, helping individuals maintain a balance between their health and their professional or academic responsibilities.

The psychological impact of CFS is also explored, with a focus on mental health challenges such as anxiety and depression. The book offers strategies for maintaining mental well-being, professional psychological support, and insights into how CFS affects relationships and social life.

The book provides an in-depth look at the long-term outlook and prognosis for individuals with CFS. It examines factors influencing prognosis, current research on long-term outcomes, and strategies for adapting to changing symptoms while planning for future health management. With detailed FAQs addressing common concerns, this book is an essential guide for understanding and managing Chronic Fatigue Syndrome, offering hope, clarity, and practical support.

CHAPTER ONE

OVERVIEW OF CHRONIC FATIGUE SYNDROME

DEFINITION

Chronic Fatigue Syndrome (CFS) is a complex and debilitating condition characterized by profound fatigue that doesn't improve with rest and worsens with physical or mental activity. The fatigue experienced is not just ordinary tiredness but a persistent exhaustion that significantly impairs daily functioning. The exact cause of CFS remains unknown, but it is believed to involve a combination of genetic, environmental, and possibly viral factors. Understanding CFS involves recognizing that it is more than just feeling tired; it is a serious condition that affects various aspects of health and quality of life.

Diagnosis of CFS is challenging due to its overlap with many other health issues. There is no definitive test for CFS, so healthcare providers rely on a combination of medical history, symptom evaluation, and the exclusion of other conditions. The diagnosis is often made based on the presence of chronic fatigue lasting more than six months, along with other specific symptoms that meet established criteria.

This process requires careful consideration and sometimes multiple evaluations to ensure an accurate diagnosis.

Management of CFS is primarily focused on relieving symptoms and improving quality of life. This may include a combination of medication, physical therapy, and lifestyle adjustments.

Individuals with CFS need to work closely with their healthcare providers to develop a personalized treatment plan that addresses their unique needs. Understanding and managing CFS effectively requires patience, support, and ongoing medical care.

The primary symptom of Chronic Fatigue Syndrome is persistent and profound fatigue that is not alleviated by rest and often worsens with physical or mental exertion. This fatigue must be present for at least six months and is typically accompanied by other symptoms.

Key symptoms include unrefreshing sleep, muscle and joint pain, headaches, sore throat, and swollen lymph nodes. Additionally, cognitive impairments, such as difficulty concentrating and memory problems, are common and can significantly impact daily functioning.

To meet the diagnostic criteria for CFS, patients must experience these symptoms consistently and to a degree that affects their ability to perform normal daily activities. The fatigue and associated symptoms should not be attributable to other medical or psychiatric conditions. Healthcare providers use specific diagnostic criteria, such as those outlined by the Centers for Disease Control and Prevention (CDC), to determine if a patient meets the requirements for a CFS diagnosis.

Evaluating the severity and impact of symptoms is crucial for developing an effective treatment plan. Healthcare providers may use questionnaires and diagnostic tools to assess the intensity and impact of fatigue and other symptoms. This information helps in tailoring treatment strategies and tracking progress over time, ensuring that the management plan remains aligned with the patient's evolving needs.

DIFFERENCE BETWEEN CFS AND OTHER FATIGUE DISORDERS

Chronic Fatigue Syndrome differs from other fatigue disorders in several ways, primarily in its persistence and the broad range of associated symptoms. Unlike general fatigue from overwork or temporary illness, CFS involves long-term fatigue that does not improve with rest and can significantly disrupt daily life.

It also presents with a combination of symptoms, such as unrefreshing sleep and cognitive impairments, that are not typically found in other fatigue-related conditions.

Other fatigue disorders, such as fibromyalgia or adrenal insufficiency, may share some symptoms with CFS but have distinct characteristics. Fibromyalgia, for example, is characterized by widespread pain and tender points, whereas CFS includes a broader range of symptoms beyond pain, including significant cognitive difficulties. Adrenal insufficiency, on the other hand, is a hormonal imbalance that can cause fatigue but is usually associated with other specific symptoms like weight loss and low blood pressure.

Proper differentiation between CFS and other conditions is crucial for effective management. Accurate diagnosis requires a thorough evaluation to rule out other potential causes of fatigue and to identify the unique features of CFS. This process helps ensure that patients receive appropriate treatment for their specific condition, improving their chances of symptom relief and better management.

IMPORTANCE OF DIAGNOSIS

Accurate diagnosis of Chronic Fatigue Syndrome is essential for several reasons. First, it helps distinguish CFS from other medical conditions with similar symptoms, ensuring that patients receive the correct treatment. Misdiagnosis can lead to inappropriate therapies and prolonged suffering, making early and precise diagnosis critical for effective management.

Additionally, a correct diagnosis allows healthcare providers to offer appropriate support and resources tailored to managing CFS. This may include specialized care, access to support groups, and strategies to manage the debilitating symptoms of CFS. Understanding the diagnosis also helps patients and their families comprehend the nature of the illness and the need for a comprehensive management plan.

Finally, an accurate diagnosis plays a role in validating the patient's experience. Since CFS is often misunderstood and sometimes dismissed, a formal diagnosis provides recognition of the condition's seriousness. This validation can be important for patients in seeking appropriate care, accessing necessary support services, and advocating for themselves within the healthcare system.

IMPACT ON DAILY LIFE

Chronic Fatigue Syndrome can have a profound impact on daily life, affecting both physical and mental well-being. The persistent fatigue and other symptoms can make routine activities challenging, leading to reduced productivity and a diminished quality of life. Individuals with CFS may find it difficult to maintain employment, manage household tasks, and engage in social or recreational activities due to the debilitating nature of their symptoms.

The cognitive impairments associated with CFS, such as memory issues and difficulty concentrating, can further complicate daily functioning. These cognitive difficulties can impact job performance, personal relationships, and the ability to perform everyday tasks. The overall effect is a significant reduction in the individual's ability to participate fully in their normal activities and responsibilities.

Additionally, the emotional and psychological impact of CFS can be considerable. The chronic nature of the condition, combined with its often invisible symptoms, can lead to feelings of frustration, isolation, and depression. Managing CFS requires not only addressing the physical symptoms but also providing emotional support and coping strategies to help individuals navigate the challenges posed by the condition.

CHAPTER TWO
MEDICAL DIAGNOSIS AND TESTING
DIAGNOSTIC CRITERIA OVERVIEW

Chronic Fatigue Syndrome (CFS) is diagnosed based on specific criteria outlined by medical guidelines. To be diagnosed with CFS, a patient must exhibit persistent fatigue that is not alleviated by rest and lasts for at least six months. This fatigue must be severe enough to significantly impair daily functioning and cannot be explained by other medical conditions. Additionally, patients often experience at least four of the following symptoms: unrefreshing sleep, muscle or joint pain, headaches, impaired memory or concentration, and post-exertional malaise that lasts more than 24 hours.

The diagnostic criteria also involve ruling out other possible causes of fatigue. This means that a comprehensive medical history and physical examination are necessary to exclude conditions such as hypothyroidism, diabetes, or depression. It is crucial to establish that the fatigue is not due to any other primary medical or psychiatric condition. This thorough evaluation helps ensure that the diagnosis of CFS is accurate and that other potential diagnoses are considered.

Medical professionals use established criteria, such as the Fukuda Criteria or the CDC's case definition, to assess whether a patient's symptoms meet the requirements for a CFS diagnosis. These criteria provide a standardized approach for evaluating symptoms and are critical in ensuring consistency in diagnosing and managing the condition across different healthcare settings.

COMMON TESTS AND PROCEDURES

Diagnosis of Chronic Fatigue Syndrome involves several tests and procedures to rule out other conditions and confirm the diagnosis. Blood tests are commonly used to check for underlying medical issues, such as anemia, thyroid function, or infections. A complete blood count (CBC) and tests for liver and kidney function can help identify other health problems that might contribute to fatigue.

In some cases, doctors may order imaging studies, such as X-rays or MRIs, to investigate any potential structural abnormalities that could be causing symptoms.

Additionally, sleep studies might be conducted if there is a suspicion of sleep disorders, such as sleep apnea, which can contribute to fatigue. These tests help to ensure that the fatigue is not due to other diagnosable conditions.

Specialized tests may be used to assess how well the body handles physical exertion. For example, exercise tolerance tests can measure how physical activity impacts fatigue and recovery. This helps differentiate CFS from other conditions with similar symptoms and provides insight into the patient's specific condition.

ROLE OF PRIMARY CARE PHYSICIANS AND SPECIALISTS

Primary care physicians play a crucial role in the initial evaluation and ongoing management of Chronic Fatigue Syndrome. They start by taking a detailed medical history and performing a physical examination to assess the patient's overall health and symptom severity. Primary care doctors often conduct initial tests to rule out other potential causes of fatigue and may refer the patient to specialists if needed.

Specialists, such as infectious disease experts, rheumatologists, or endocrinologists, are often consulted for a more in-depth evaluation. These specialists can provide targeted tests and treatment options based on their area of expertise. For example, a rheumatologist might be involved if there is a suspected overlap with autoimmune conditions, while an infectious disease specialist might be consulted if there is a history of viral infections.

Collaboration between primary care physicians and specialists is essential for comprehensive care. Effective communication ensures that all aspects of the patient's health are considered, and a coordinated approach to diagnosis and treatment is achieved. This teamwork helps to manage symptoms and improve the quality of life for individuals with CFS.

INTERPRETING TEST RESULTS

Interpreting test results in Chronic Fatigue Syndrome requires careful consideration of the patient's symptoms and overall health. Blood tests and imaging studies should be reviewed to rule out other conditions and confirm that no underlying health issues are contributing to the fatigue. It's important to analyze the results in the context of the patient's clinical presentation and not in isolation.

Healthcare providers use test results to differentiate Chronic Fatigue Syndrome from other similar conditions. For example, normal blood test results and imaging studies can support the diagnosis of CFS when other potential causes of fatigue are excluded. Understanding the results involves correlating them with the patient's symptoms, such as persistent fatigue and unrefreshing sleep.

Effective interpretation also involves considering any abnormalities in test results that may indicate other health issues. For instance, slight abnormalities in thyroid function tests may prompt further evaluation for thyroid disorders.

Accurate interpretation helps in refining the diagnosis and guiding appropriate treatment strategies for managing Chronic Fatigue Syndrome.

STEPS TO OBTAIN A DIAGNOSIS

To obtain a diagnosis of Chronic Fatigue Syndrome, patients typically start by consulting their primary care physician. The process begins with a detailed medical history and physical examination to evaluate symptoms and rule out other conditions. The physician may then order initial tests to exclude common causes of fatigue, such as infections or metabolic disorders.

If the initial evaluation suggests the possibility of CFS, the patient may be referred to a specialist for further assessment. Specialists can conduct more specific tests, such as sleep studies or exercise tolerance tests, to confirm the diagnosis. This step is crucial for differentiating CFS from other similar conditions and ensuring an accurate diagnosis.

Once a diagnosis of Chronic Fatigue Syndrome is made, the focus shifts to developing a management plan. This plan may include lifestyle modifications, symptom management strategies, and referrals to support services. Continuous follow-up with healthcare providers helps to monitor progress, adjust treatment plans, and provide ongoing support for managing the condition effectively.

CHAPTER THREE

TREATMENT OPTIONS AND MANAGEMENT

OVERVIEW OF TREATMENT APPROACHES

Chronic Fatigue Syndrome (CFS) treatment is multifaceted, focusing on alleviating symptoms and improving quality of life. The primary goal is to reduce fatigue and associated symptoms such as sleep disturbances and cognitive difficulties. Treatment approaches typically involve a combination of medications, lifestyle changes, and various therapies tailored to individual needs. Due to the complex nature of CFS, a multidisciplinary approach often works best, involving primary care physicians, specialists, and therapists who can collaboratively address different aspects of the condition.

The effectiveness of treatments can vary from person to person, and ongoing adjustments may be necessary. For some, the use of a structured management plan, which includes symptom tracking and regular follow-up visits, can help in fine-tuning treatments. This approach allows healthcare providers to make informed decisions about adjusting or combining treatments to achieve the best outcomes. It is also essential to educate patients about the nature of CFS, which helps in setting realistic expectations and encourages adherence to the treatment plan.

Monitoring progress is crucial in the management of CFS. Regular evaluations help assess the effectiveness of the treatment and make necessary adjustments. Utilizing symptom diaries and other tracking tools can be beneficial for both patients and healthcare providers. This ongoing assessment ensures that the treatment plan remains aligned with the patient's evolving needs and helps in managing any new symptoms that may arise.

MEDICATIONS AND SUPPLEMENTS

Medications for CFS primarily aim to manage symptoms rather than cure the condition. Commonly prescribed medications include pain relievers, antidepressants, and sleep aids. Pain relievers, such as ibuprofen or acetaminophen, can help with muscle and joint pain. Antidepressants may be used to address both mood disorders and sleep issues, which are prevalent in CFS patients. It's important to work closely with a healthcare provider to select the right medication and dosage, as individual responses can vary.

Supplements, including vitamins and minerals, may also play a role in managing CFS symptoms. Some patients benefit from taking supplements like vitamin B12, magnesium, or omega-3 fatty acids, which can support overall health and potentially improve energy levels. Before starting any supplement regimen, it is essential to consult with a healthcare provider to ensure that the supplements are appropriate and do not interact with other medications or conditions.

Regular monitoring and adjustments are necessary when using medications and supplements. Patients should report any side effects or changes in symptoms to their healthcare provider. This helps in fine-tuning the treatment plan and ensuring that the chosen medications and supplements are contributing positively to the management of CFS.

LIFESTYLE MODIFICATIONS

Lifestyle changes are crucial in managing CFS and can significantly impact overall well-being. Pacing oneself is a fundamental strategy, involving balancing activity with rest to avoid exacerbating fatigue. This often means breaking tasks into smaller, manageable steps and incorporating regular periods of rest. Creating a consistent daily routine can help in managing energy levels and preventing overexertion.

Diet and nutrition play a significant role in managing CFS. Eating a balanced diet rich in fruits, vegetables, lean proteins, and whole grains can support overall health and energy levels. Staying hydrated is equally important, as dehydration can worsen fatigue. Regular, moderate exercise, tailored to individual capacity, can also be beneficial, as it helps in maintaining physical fitness and improving energy levels over time.

Sleep hygiene is another essential aspect of lifestyle modification. Establishing a regular sleep schedule and creating a restful environment can improve sleep quality, which is often disrupted in CFS patients. Techniques such as avoiding stimulants before bedtime, maintaining a cool and dark sleeping area, and practicing relaxation exercises can help enhance sleep and, consequently, manage fatigue more effectively.

COGNITIVE-BEHAVIORAL THERAPY (CBT) AND OTHER THERAPIES

Cognitive-behavioral therapy (CBT) is a well-established approach for managing CFS and addressing the psychological aspects of the condition. CBT helps patients identify and change negative thought patterns and behaviors that may contribute to their fatigue and stress. Through structured sessions with a trained therapist, patients learn coping strategies and problem-solving skills that can improve their overall quality of life.

Other therapeutic options may include graded exercise therapy (GET), which involves gradually increasing physical activity levels in a controlled manner.

This approach aims to improve physical fitness and reduce symptoms over time. Patients work with a therapist to develop an exercise plan that is tailored to their specific needs and capabilities, ensuring that they do not overexert themselves.

In addition to CBT and GET, patients may benefit from complementary therapies such as mindfulness and relaxation techniques. These approaches can help in managing stress and improving mental well-being, which can, in turn, alleviate some of the symptoms associated with CFS. Integrating these therapies into the overall treatment plan can enhance the effectiveness of other treatment modalities.

MANAGING COEXISTING CONDITIONS

Managing coexisting conditions is an integral part of treating CFS, as these conditions can exacerbate fatigue and other symptoms. Common coexisting conditions include fibromyalgia, irritable bowel syndrome (IBS), and sleep disorders. Addressing these conditions requires a comprehensive approach, involving both symptom management and treatment of the underlying issues.

Treatment strategies for coexisting conditions often include specific medications, dietary changes, and targeted therapies. For example, managing IBS might involve dietary modifications and medications to control digestive symptoms, while fibromyalgia might be treated with pain management techniques and physical therapy.

It is important to coordinate care with healthcare providers who are knowledgeable about these conditions to ensure an integrated treatment approach.

Regular follow-up and communication with healthcare providers are essential in managing coexisting conditions. Patients should actively report any changes in symptoms or new issues that arise, as this information is crucial for adjusting treatment plans and improving overall management. By addressing all aspects of their health, patients with CFS can achieve better symptom control and an improved quality of life.

CHAPTER FOUR

SELF-CARE AND LIFESTYLE ADJUSTMENTS

IMPORTANCE OF SELF-CARE ROUTINES

Implementing self-care routines is essential for managing Chronic Fatigue Syndrome (CFS) effectively. These routines help in maintaining balance and managing symptoms by incorporating activities that enhance overall well-being.

Prioritizing self-care involves setting aside time for relaxation and activities that promote physical and mental health, such as hobbies or mindfulness practices. Consistency is key, as regular self-care helps in stabilizing energy levels and reducing the impact of fatigue.

Establishing a structured routine can significantly improve daily functioning. Create a schedule that includes time for self-care activities, ensuring these practices become a natural part of your day. For instance, integrating short breaks during work, practicing deep breathing exercises, or engaging in relaxing activities like reading can provide respite and recharge energy levels. The goal is to create a balance that accommodates both activity and rest, reducing the likelihood of burnout.

Personalizing self-care routines to fit individual needs is crucial. Identify activities that bring joy and relaxation and make them a regular part of your day. It's also beneficial to periodically reassess and adjust these routines based on how your symptoms fluctuate. A well-balanced self-care routine tailored to your preferences and energy levels can significantly alleviate the symptoms of CFS and improve your overall quality of life.

DIETARY RECOMMENDATIONS

A well-balanced diet plays a critical role in managing Chronic Fatigue Syndrome. Emphasize nutrient-dense foods that support energy levels and overall health. Incorporate a variety of fruits, vegetables, whole grains, lean proteins, and healthy fats into your meals. Foods rich in antioxidants, vitamins, and minerals can help combat inflammation and support immune function, which is beneficial for those with CFS.

Monitoring and managing food intake can further aid in reducing fatigue. Consider eating smaller, more frequent meals to maintain stable blood sugar levels and avoid energy crashes.

Additionally, staying hydrated is vital, so aim to drink plenty of water throughout the day. Limiting caffeine and processed foods can also help in managing symptoms more effectively, as these can contribute to fluctuations in energy levels and overall health.

Consulting with a registered dietitian can provide personalized dietary guidance tailored to your specific needs. A dietitian can help in developing a meal plan that aligns with your energy levels and nutritional requirements. This professional support can be invaluable in ensuring you're making the right food choices to manage CFS and enhance your overall health.

EXERCISE AND PHYSICAL ACTIVITY GUIDELINES

Incorporating exercise into your routine can help manage Chronic Fatigue Syndrome, but it must be approached with caution. Start with low-impact activities such as walking, stretching, or gentle yoga to avoid overexertion.

Gradually increase the intensity and duration of exercise based on your tolerance and energy levels. Aim to engage in physical activity for short periods, focusing on consistency rather than intensity to avoid exacerbating symptoms.

Pay attention to your body's signals and adjust your activity levels accordingly. It's important to balance exercise with adequate rest to prevent fatigue from worsening. Establishing a regular, moderate exercise routine can help improve stamina and reduce symptoms over time. Listening to your body and making adjustments based on how you feel will help in maintaining a manageable exercise routine without overwhelming yourself.

Incorporating exercise as part of a comprehensive management plan can enhance physical fitness and contribute to overall well-being. Working with a healthcare provider or physical therapist can provide additional guidance on developing a safe and effective exercise program tailored to your specific needs.

This professional support can help ensure that your exercise routine complements your self-care and dietary efforts effectively.

STRESS MANAGEMENT TECHNIQUES

Effective stress management is crucial for individuals with Chronic Fatigue Syndrome, as stress can exacerbate symptoms and hinder recovery. Incorporate techniques such as deep breathing exercises, meditation, or progressive muscle relaxation into your daily routine.

These methods can help calm the mind and reduce physical tension, leading to improved overall well-being and energy levels.

Engaging in activities that bring joy and relaxation can also help manage stress. Consider hobbies, socializing with supportive friends, or spending time in nature as ways to alleviate stress. Establishing boundaries and prioritizing time for self-care can prevent overwhelm and maintain a balanced lifestyle. Regularly practicing these stress-relief techniques can help in managing the emotional and physical impacts of CFS more effectively.

It's beneficial to identify and address specific stressors that may contribute to your symptoms. Working with a mental health professional can provide additional support and strategies for managing stress. Developing personalized stress management techniques in collaboration with a professional can enhance your ability to cope with the demands of CFS and improve your overall quality of life.

SLEEP HYGIENE PRACTICES

Good sleep hygiene is essential for managing Chronic Fatigue Syndrome, as quality sleep directly impacts energy levels and overall health. Establish a consistent sleep schedule by going to bed and waking up at the same time each day. Create a relaxing bedtime routine that helps signal to your body that it's time to wind down, such as reading a book or taking a warm bath.

Optimize your sleep environment to promote restful sleep. Ensure your bedroom is cool, dark, and quiet, and invest in a comfortable mattress and pillows. Limiting screen time before bed and avoiding stimulants like caffeine can help improve sleep quality. Making these adjustments can enhance your ability to fall asleep and stay asleep, which is crucial for managing fatigue and promoting recovery.

If sleep problems persist despite good sleep hygiene practices, consider consulting a healthcare provider for further evaluation.

They can help identify any underlying sleep disorders or provide additional recommendations tailored to your needs. Effective management of sleep quality is a key component in alleviating the symptoms of CFS and improving overall well-being.

CHAPTER FIVE

BUILDING A SUPPORT NETWORK

FINDING SUPPORT GROUPS

Finding a support group for Chronic Fatigue Syndrome (CFS) involves researching local and national organizations dedicated to the condition. Start by looking for groups through reputable health organizations such as the Chronic Fatigue Syndrome Association or similar entities.

These groups often provide directories or listings of support groups, which can be accessed via their websites or contact numbers. Attending local health fairs or medical clinics can also help identify in-person support group meetings where you can connect with others facing similar challenges.

Once you have identified potential support groups, consider attending a few sessions to see which one best meets your needs. Look for groups with a structured approach, facilitated by experienced leaders who understand the nuances of CFS. Participation in these groups can offer valuable emotional support, practical advice on managing symptoms, and an opportunity to share experiences with others who truly understand the condition. Many support groups also offer guest speakers, educational workshops, and the chance to build lasting connections with others in similar situations.

It is also beneficial to check if the support groups offer virtual meetings. Online options can provide greater flexibility and accessibility, especially if mobility or geographic constraints are an issue. Join these groups to benefit from a wider network of individuals and resources. Engaging in both local and online support groups can provide a comprehensive support system that helps manage the complexities of living with CFS.

INVOLVING FAMILY AND FRIENDS

Involving family and friends in your journey with Chronic Fatigue Syndrome is crucial for creating a supportive environment. Begin by having open and honest conversations about the condition, explaining the symptoms and challenges you face. This helps them understand the impact of CFS on your daily life and how they can best offer support. Share specific ways they can assist, such as helping with household chores, providing emotional support, or accommodating your need for rest.

Encourage your loved ones to educate themselves about CFS through reputable resources. This can help them empathize with your experiences and adjust their expectations accordingly.

Provide them with information from credible sources, such as medical professionals or patient advocacy organizations, to enhance their understanding and support. Involving family and friends in learning about CFS fosters a more compassionate and informed support network.

Regular communication with family and friends is essential to address any misunderstandings or adjustments needed as your condition evolves. Schedule periodic discussions to review how things are going and what additional support might be necessary. This ongoing dialogue ensures that your support system remains responsive to your needs and can adapt as your situation changes.

PROFESSIONAL COUNSELING AND THERAPY

Professional counseling and therapy play a significant role in managing Chronic Fatigue Syndrome. Start by consulting a healthcare provider who can refer you to a therapist with experience in chronic illness and fatigue management. Cognitive-behavioral therapy (CBT) is commonly used to help individuals with CFS by addressing negative thought patterns and developing coping strategies. Engage actively in therapy sessions to explore emotional challenges and learn techniques to manage stress and fatigue.

Therapists can also offer valuable insights into managing symptoms and improving quality of life through personalized strategies.

They may help you set realistic goals, develop a balanced routine, and identify triggers that exacerbate symptoms. Consistent therapy sessions can provide ongoing support, helping you to build resilience and adapt to the demands of living with CFS.

Additionally, therapists can facilitate group therapy sessions, where individuals with similar conditions come together to share experiences and strategies. This can offer a sense of community and shared understanding, further enhancing your support network. Regular engagement in therapy can significantly contribute to managing both the emotional and practical aspects of CFS.

Online communities and resources are invaluable for individuals with Chronic Fatigue Syndrome seeking support and information. Begin by exploring forums and social media groups dedicated to CFS. These platforms provide a space for individuals to share their experiences, seek advice, and offer support to one another. Engage in discussions to gain insights and strategies from others who understand the condition firsthand.

Look for reputable online resources that offer educational materials, symptom management tips, and updates on research related to CFS. Websites of organizations such as the Centers for Disease Control and Prevention (CDC) or specialized CFS foundations provide credible information and can guide you to additional resources. Bookmark these sites for easy access to up-to-date information and useful tools.

Participate in webinars, virtual support groups, and online workshops hosted by CFS organizations. These events offer opportunities to learn from experts, connect with others in similar situations, and stay informed about new developments in CFS research and treatment. Utilizing online communities and resources can enhance your understanding of the condition and provide continuous support.

ADVOCACY AND RAISING AWARENESS

Advocacy and raising awareness for Chronic Fatigue Syndrome are essential for improving public understanding and support. Start by getting involved with local or national CFS advocacy organizations. These groups often campaign for better research funding, healthcare access, and public awareness. Participate in events, sign petitions, and support their initiatives to amplify the voice of those affected by CFS.

Utilize social media platforms to share your personal experiences with CFS, educating your network about the challenges and needs of individuals living with the condition. By sharing stories and information, you can help dispel myths, increase awareness, and foster a more supportive community. Encourage friends and family to do the same to broaden the impact.

Engage in or organize community events such as fundraisers, awareness walks, or informational seminars.

These activities can raise funds for research and support services while also educating the public about CFS. Active participation in advocacy efforts helps build a stronger support system and drives progress in addressing the needs of those with Chronic Fatigue Syndrome.

CHAPTER SIX

NAVIGATING THE HEALTHCARE SYSTEM

WORKING WITH HEALTHCARE PROVIDERS

When navigating the healthcare system for Chronic Fatigue Syndrome (CFS), establishing a strong relationship with healthcare providers is crucial. Start by finding a specialist familiar with CFS, such as a rheumatologist or an infectious disease expert, as they can offer targeted treatments and advice. Prepare for appointments by documenting your symptoms, medical history, and any treatments you've tried. This preparation helps your provider understand your condition better and develop a tailored treatment plan. Ensure open communication by asking questions about treatment options, potential side effects, and expected outcomes.

During consultations, actively participate by expressing your concerns and preferences. Make sure to keep track of the advice and instructions given, and don't hesitate to ask for clarification if needed. It's important to follow the recommended treatment plans and adhere to prescribed medications to manage CFS effectively. Regular follow-ups with your provider are essential for monitoring progress and adjusting treatment as necessary. Building a collaborative relationship with your healthcare team can significantly impact your overall management of the condition.

In addition, seek out healthcare providers who take a holistic approach to treatment. This might include integrating lifestyle changes, such as dietary adjustments and stress management techniques, into your care plan. A provider who recognizes the complexity of CFS and is willing to explore various treatment avenues will be more effective in supporting your journey toward better health. Always ensure that your healthcare team is updated about any changes in your condition or response to treatments.

UNDERSTANDING INSURANCE AND COVERAGE

Navigating insurance and coverage for CFS treatment involves understanding your policy details and how they apply to your care. Begin by reviewing your health insurance plan to identify what is covered, such as specialist visits, diagnostic tests, and medications.

Look for specific terms related to chronic illness management, and note any limitations or exclusions that may affect your coverage. Contact your insurance provider to clarify any doubts and ensure you understand the benefits and limitations of your plan.

Understanding your policy's coverage for CFS treatment is crucial for avoiding unexpected expenses. Some insurance plans may require pre-authorization for certain treatments or referrals to specialists. Make sure to get all necessary approvals before proceeding with treatments to ensure coverage. Keep detailed records of all interactions with your insurance company, including phone calls, emails, and written correspondence, to manage any disputes or claims efficiently.

Additionally, explore options for financial assistance if your insurance does not cover all aspects of your care. This may include applying for patient assistance programs offered by pharmaceutical companies or seeking help from non-profit organizations dedicated to chronic illness support.

Being proactive and informed about your insurance coverage will help you manage the financial aspects of your CFS treatment effectively.

SEEKING SECOND OPINIONS

Obtaining a second opinion can be a valuable step in managing CFS, especially if you have doubts about your initial diagnosis or treatment plan. Start by gathering all relevant medical records and test results from your primary healthcare provider. Then, consult with another specialist who has experience with CFS to review your case.

Provide them with all necessary documentation and discuss your current treatment plan and symptoms in detail.

When seeking a second opinion, it's important to choose a specialist who is knowledgeable about CFS and can offer a fresh perspective on your condition. This might involve visiting a different healthcare facility or consulting with a specialist who uses alternative diagnostic approaches. The goal is to gain additional insights that may lead to a more effective treatment strategy or confirm the validity of your current plan.

After receiving the second opinion, compare the recommendations with your original treatment plan. This comparison can help you make informed decisions about your care and potentially incorporate new strategies that could improve your management of CFS. Remember that a second opinion is a tool to empower you in your healthcare journey and ensure that you are receiving the best possible care.

MANAGING MEDICAL APPOINTMENTS

Effectively managing medical appointments is key to navigating the complexities of CFS treatment. Start by keeping a detailed calendar or planner to track all scheduled appointments, tests, and follow-ups. This organization helps prevent missed appointments and ensures that you stay on top of your healthcare needs. Set reminders for each appointment and prepare in advance by gathering any required documents or medical history.

During appointments, make the most of your time with healthcare providers by coming prepared with a list of questions and concerns. Take notes during the visit to remember important details and instructions given by your provider.

If possible, bring a friend or family member to help with note-taking and provide support. Managing appointments efficiently ensures that you adhere to your treatment plan and stay informed about your condition.

Follow up on any additional actions required after your appointments, such as scheduling further tests or referrals to other specialists. Ensure that you understand the next steps and any changes to your treatment plan. Proper management of your medical appointments helps maintain continuity of care and supports better overall management of CFS.

ADVOCATING FOR YOURSELF IN MEDICAL SETTINGS

Self-advocacy in medical settings is essential for effective CFS management. Begin by being well-informed about your condition and treatment options. Educate yourself about CFS through reputable sources and discuss any relevant information with your healthcare provider. Communicate your symptoms, concerns, and treatment preferences to ensure that your needs are addressed.

Assertiveness is key when advocating for yourself. Don't hesitate to ask questions, request clarifications, and express your concerns if you feel that your treatment plan isn't meeting your needs. If you encounter obstacles or disagreements, remain calm and persistent in seeking resolutions. Documenting your interactions and maintaining open communication with your healthcare team can help facilitate better outcomes.

Additionally, seek support from patient advocacy organizations or support groups for CFS. These resources can provide valuable information, share experiences, and offer guidance on navigating medical settings. Empowering yourself through knowledge and support enhances your ability to advocate effectively and ensures that you receive appropriate care for your condition.

CHAPTER SEVEN

WORK AND EDUCATION CONSIDERATIONS

MANAGING CFS IN THE WORKPLACE

Managing Chronic Fatigue Syndrome (CFS) in the workplace involves a multi-faceted approach tailored to the individual's needs.

This includes establishing a flexible work schedule that accommodates periods of rest and reduces the risk of overexertion. Employees must communicate their condition to their supervisors or HR departments to ensure understanding and support. Implementing a gradual return-to-work plan can help ease the transition and prevent exacerbation of symptoms.

Adapting the work environment is also key. This might involve ergonomic adjustments, such as a more comfortable chair or desk setup, to minimize physical strain. Reducing workplace stressors by allowing for breaks and providing a quiet area for rest can further help manage fatigue. Additionally, ensuring that workload expectations are realistic and manageable is vital to prevent burnout.

Employees should actively engage in self-care practices and use available resources to manage their condition. This includes utilizing productivity tools and techniques designed for people with chronic conditions, such as time management apps that schedule rest periods.

Regularly assessing and adjusting the work environment and schedule based on feedback can lead to better management of CFS and improved workplace well-being.

LEGAL RIGHTS AND ACCOMMODATIONS

Understanding legal rights and accommodations for individuals with CFS is essential to ensure they receive the necessary support at work. Under laws such as the Americans with Disabilities Act (ADA) in the U.S., individuals with CFS are entitled to reasonable accommodations. These accommodations might include adjustments to work hours, modifications to job duties, or provision of special equipment to aid in daily tasks.

Employers are required to engage in an interactive process to determine appropriate accommodations. This involves discussions between the employee and employer to identify specific needs and possible adjustments. Employees need to provide medical documentation to support their request for accommodations and to advocate for their rights if necessary.

Employees should be aware of their legal protections and seek assistance from advocacy groups or legal advisors if they face resistance or denial of reasonable accommodations. Knowing one's rights ensures that individuals with CFS can effectively navigate the workplace and obtain the support they need to perform their jobs effectively.

BALANCING WORK AND HEALTH

Balancing work and health with CFS requires careful planning and self-management. It involves setting realistic goals and prioritizing tasks based on energy levels. Employees should develop a daily schedule that includes regular breaks and time for rest to prevent overexertion. Monitoring energy levels and adjusting work activities accordingly can help maintain a balance between productivity and health.

Time management techniques, such as breaking tasks into smaller, manageable chunks and using tools like planners or digital calendars, can help manage workload without overwhelming oneself. Establishing boundaries between work and personal life is also crucial to avoid burnout. This might include setting clear work hours and ensuring time off for rest and recovery.

Engaging in regular communication with supervisors and colleagues about one's needs and limitations can foster a supportive work environment.

Flexibility and understanding from both sides can enhance the ability to balance work and health, making it easier to manage CFS effectively while fulfilling job responsibilities.

EDUCATIONAL SUPPORT AND ACCOMMODATIONS

Educational support and accommodations for students with CFS are vital to ensure they can participate fully in their learning environment. This might involve modifications to the physical environment, such as allowing for rest periods or providing a quiet space for studying.

Teachers and educational institutions need to be informed about the student's condition to tailor support effectively.

Accommodations may include flexible deadlines, modified coursework, and alternative methods of assessment. Implementing a plan that allows for adjustments based on the student's fluctuating energy levels can help manage academic demands without exacerbating symptoms. Collaboration between students, parents, and educators is essential to create an effective support system.

Students with CFS should advocate for themselves and communicate their needs clearly to educators. Utilizing support services offered by educational institutions, such as counseling or academic advising, can also provide additional assistance.

A proactive approach to seeking and managing accommodations can lead to a more manageable and successful educational experience.

STRATEGIES FOR PRODUCTIVITY AND ENERGY MANAGEMENT

Developing strategies for productivity and energy management is crucial for individuals with CFS to maintain efficiency while managing their condition. Prioritizing tasks based on importance and energy levels helps ensure that the most critical work is completed when energy is highest.

Utilizing tools such as to-do lists and scheduling apps can aid in organizing tasks and avoiding overwhelm?

Energy management techniques, such as pacing oneself and incorporating rest periods into the daily routine, are essential. The use of time-blocking methods, where specific periods are allocated for work and rest, can help manage energy more effectively. It's also beneficial to identify and minimize factors that contribute to fatigue, such as excessive stress or poor ergonomics.

Regular evaluation and adjustment of productivity strategies based on personal experiences and feedback can lead to improved outcomes. Experimenting with different techniques and remaining flexible in approach allows individuals to find what works best for managing their energy levels and maintaining productivity over time.

CHAPTER EIGHT

PSYCHOLOGICAL IMPACT AND SUPPORT

ADDRESSING MENTAL HEALTH CHALLENGES

Chronic Fatigue Syndrome (CFS) can significantly affect mental health, often leading to heightened stress and emotional strain.

Addressing these challenges begins with recognizing the symptoms and understanding their impact on one's mental well-being. Individuals with CFS may experience feelings of helplessness or frustration due to their limited energy levels, which can exacerbate existing mental health issues. It's crucial to acknowledge these emotions as a legitimate part of the condition and not just a result of the fatigue itself.

One practical approach to addressing these mental health challenges is to incorporate structured routines and goal-setting. Establishing small, achievable goals can help manage the overwhelming nature of CFS.

Setting up a daily schedule that balances rest with light activities can create a sense of control and accomplishment. This method can alleviate feelings of helplessness and provide a framework for managing the unpredictability of CFS symptoms.

Support systems also play a vital role in tackling mental health challenges. Engaging with support groups or counseling services can provide a safe space for individuals to express their emotions and share experiences with others facing similar difficulties. These interactions can foster a sense of community and understanding, which is essential for emotional support and resilience.

COPING WITH ANXIETY AND DEPRESSION

Anxiety and depression are common among those with Chronic Fatigue Syndrome, and effective coping strategies are essential for managing these conditions. One fundamental technique is mindfulness and relaxation exercises, such as deep breathing, meditation, or progressive muscle relaxation. These practices can help calm the mind, reduce anxiety, and improve mood, offering relief from the mental strain associated with CFS.

Another effective coping strategy involves cognitive-behavioral techniques that address negative thought patterns. Engaging in therapy sessions that focus on challenging and changing unhelpful thoughts can be particularly beneficial. Keeping a journal to track feelings and thoughts can also help identify triggers and patterns, allowing individuals to develop more constructive coping mechanisms over time.

Additionally, integrating physical activity within the limits of one's energy can also be helpful. Gentle exercises, like stretching or short walks, can improve mood and reduce symptoms of depression.

STRATEGIES FOR MAINTAINING MENTAL WELL-BEING

Maintaining mental well-being in the context of Chronic Fatigue Syndrome involves developing a balanced lifestyle that incorporates self-care and stress management. Regular sleep patterns are crucial, as adequate rest can improve both physical and mental health. Establishing a consistent sleep schedule and creating a restful environment can enhance sleep quality and overall well-being.

Healthy eating habits also play a role in sustaining mental health. A balanced diet rich in nutrients supports brain function and mood regulation. Individuals with CFS should focus on consuming a variety of fruits, vegetables, whole grains, and proteins while avoiding excessive caffeine and sugar, which can impact energy levels and mood stability.

Routine self-care activities, such as engaging in hobbies, spending time in nature, or practicing relaxation techniques, can provide emotional relief and improve mental health.

PROFESSIONAL PSYCHOLOGICAL SUPPORT

Seeking professional psychological support is often necessary for managing the mental health aspects of

Chronic Fatigue Syndrome. Therapy with a licensed mental health professional can provide a structured approach to addressing psychological symptoms and developing coping strategies. Cognitive-behavioral therapy (CBT) is one such approach that can help individuals reframe negative thought patterns and manage stress more effectively.

Additionally, psychotherapy can offer personalized strategies for dealing with the unique challenges of CFS. A therapist can work with individuals to develop tailored coping mechanisms, set realistic goals, and provide ongoing support. Regular sessions can also serve as a valuable source of encouragement and accountability.

Medication may also be considered in some cases, especially if anxiety or depression is significantly impacting daily functioning. A healthcare provider can evaluate the need for medication, discuss potential benefits and side effects, and monitor its effectiveness in conjunction with other therapeutic interventions.

IMPACT ON RELATIONSHIPS AND SOCIAL LIFE

Chronic Fatigue Syndrome can affect relationships and social interactions, leading to feelings of isolation and strain on personal connections. Open communication with family and friends about the condition is crucial for fostering understanding and support. Sharing information about the nature of CFS can help others empathize with the limitations and challenges faced.

Maintaining social connections, despite the limitations imposed by CFS, is important for emotional support. Engaging in low-energy social activities, such as video calls or small gatherings, can help preserve relationships without overwhelming one's energy reserves. It's also beneficial to discuss one's needs and limitations with friends and family to create a supportive environment.

CHAPTER NINE

LONG-TERM OUTLOOK AND PROGNOSIS

UNDERSTANDING THE CHRONIC NATURE OF CFS

Chronic Fatigue Syndrome (CFS) is a debilitating condition characterized by persistent, unexplained fatigue that doesn't improve with rest and worsens with physical or mental exertion. This chronic nature means that individuals often experience an ongoing, fluctuating level of fatigue that can severely impact their daily functioning and quality of life. Unlike temporary fatigue, CFS can last for months or even years, affecting multiple systems in the body, including the immune system, endocrine system, and nervous system.

Patients with CFS often struggle with a range of symptoms beyond fatigue, such as cognitive impairments, sleep disturbances, and muscle or joint pain. The unpredictability of these symptoms adds to the complexity of managing the condition, as patients may experience periods of relative improvement followed by sudden relapses. Effective management requires a comprehensive approach that addresses both physical and psychological aspects of the condition, focusing on improving the patient's overall well-being and functional capacity.

Understanding the chronic nature of CFS involves recognizing that it is not a temporary or easily curable illness but a long-term health challenge. This perspective helps patients, caregivers, and healthcare providers set realistic goals and expectations, plan appropriate treatments, and develop coping strategies to manage the daily impacts of the syndrome effectively.

FACTORS INFLUENCING PROGNOSIS

The prognosis for CFS can vary widely among individuals and is influenced by a range of factors. Key determinants include the severity and duration of symptoms at onset, the presence of other coexisting health conditions, and the individual's overall health status. Early intervention and appropriate management strategies can play a significant role in influencing the long-term outlook, potentially improving symptom control and quality of life.

Lifestyle factors such as stress management, physical activity levels, and adherence to treatment plans also impact prognosis. Patients who can balance rest with gradually monitored physical activity and effectively manage stress may experience better long-term outcomes.

Additionally, a supportive social network and mental health care can contribute positively to the prognosis by providing emotional support and coping mechanisms.

Research indicates that while some individuals with CFS may experience significant improvement or remission, others may continue to have persistent symptoms. Factors such as timely diagnosis, personalized treatment approaches, and patient engagement in their care can all contribute to better management and potentially more favorable long-term outcomes.

RESEARCH ON LONG-TERM OUTCOMES

Research on CFS has explored various aspects of long-term outcomes, focusing on how the condition progresses over time and the factors that contribute to improvement or deterioration. Studies often examine the impact of different treatment modalities, lifestyle changes, and support systems on patients' long-term health.

Findings suggest that while some individuals may experience partial or full recovery, many continue to face ongoing challenges related to fatigue and other symptoms.

Long-term outcome studies emphasize the importance of individualized treatment plans that address the unique needs of each patient. Research highlights the benefits of a multidisciplinary approach, including medical care, psychological support, and lifestyle modifications. Ongoing research aims to identify predictors of better outcomes and to refine treatment strategies based on emerging evidence.

Understanding the long-term outcomes of CFS helps patients and healthcare providers make informed decisions about treatment and management. By staying abreast of current research findings, individuals with CFS can better navigate their health journey and engage in practices that may enhance their overall well-being and functional capacity.

ADAPTING TO CHANGING SYMPTOMS

CFS is characterized by fluctuating symptoms, making it crucial for patients to adapt their management strategies as their condition evolves. Adapting to changing symptoms involves recognizing patterns in symptom flare-ups and employing flexible approaches to manage them effectively. This may include adjusting daily activities, modifying treatment plans, or incorporating new coping strategies based on current symptom severity and impact.

Effective adaptation also requires regular communication with healthcare providers to reassess and adjust treatment plans as needed. Patients should be encouraged to monitor their symptoms, document any changes, and discuss these with their healthcare team to ensure that their management plan remains aligned with their current needs. Implementing strategies such as pacing, stress management, and cognitive behavioral techniques can help patients navigate the variability of their condition.

Building resilience and maintaining a proactive approach to symptom management is essential for coping with the dynamic nature of CFS. By staying informed about their condition and engaging in adaptive strategies, individuals with CFS can better manage their symptoms and improve their overall quality of life.

PLANNING FOR FUTURE HEALTH MANAGEMENT

Planning for future health management in CFS involves developing a long-term strategy to address ongoing symptoms and adapt to potential changes in the condition.

This includes setting realistic health goals, identifying resources for support, and creating a comprehensive management plan that incorporates medical care, lifestyle adjustments, and self-care practices.

A proactive approach to health management involves regular follow-ups with healthcare providers to review and update treatment plans based on the patient's evolving needs. Patients should also consider exploring complementary therapies, joining support groups, and staying informed about new research and treatment options that could benefit their condition.

Effective planning helps individuals with CFS to navigate the complexities of their condition, anticipate potential challenges, and develop strategies to maintain their well-being over the long term. By adopting a forward-thinking mindset and staying engaged in their care, patients can better manage their health and improve their overall quality of life.

CHAPTER TEN

COMMON CONCERNS AND DETAILED FAQS

WHAT IS CHRONIC FATIGUE SYNDROME AND HOW IS IT DIFFERENT FROM REGULAR FATIGUE?

Chronic Fatigue Syndrome (CFS), also known as Myalgic Encephalomyelitis (ME), is a complex and debilitating condition characterized by persistent, unexplained fatigue that does not improve with rest. Unlike regular fatigue, which typically results from overexertion or lack of sleep and resolves with rest, CFS involves profound and disabling tiredness that can be worsened by physical or mental exertion. This fatigue is often accompanied by other symptoms such as unrefreshing sleep, muscle and joint pain, and cognitive impairments, which collectively interfere with daily functioning.

The distinguishing feature of CFS is its impact on quality of life, with symptoms persisting for at least six months and leading to significant reductions in the ability to perform routine activities.

Regular fatigue, on the other hand, usually resolves with lifestyle changes such as improved sleep or stress management. CFS also differs in that it is often triggered by an initial viral infection or other stressors, but the exact cause remains unclear and may involve a combination of genetic, environmental, and physiological factors.

Understanding the difference between CFS and regular fatigue is crucial for proper diagnosis and management. While regular fatigue is often transient and can be addressed with lifestyle adjustments, CFS requires a more comprehensive approach to address its chronic nature and multi-faceted symptoms. Proper identification of CFS helps in differentiating it from other conditions with similar symptoms, ensuring appropriate treatment and support.

HOW IS CFS DIAGNOSED?

Diagnosing Chronic Fatigue Syndrome is a challenging process due to its complex and often overlapping symptoms with other medical conditions. The diagnosis typically involves a thorough medical history and a series of tests to rule out other possible causes of fatigue. This includes evaluating the patient's history of illness, current symptoms, and any previous health issues that might contribute to the fatigue.

There are no definitive tests for CFS; therefore, diagnosis is largely based on the exclusion of other medical conditions and the presence of specific criteria. Healthcare providers use diagnostic criteria such as the Fukuda or the Canadian Consensus Criteria, which require a combination of persistent fatigue, unrefreshing sleep, and a range of other symptoms, including cognitive impairment and musculoskeletal pain. The process often involves multiple visits and consultations with specialists to ensure a comprehensive evaluation.

Patients need to provide detailed information about their symptoms and how they impact their daily lives. This helps healthcare professionals to differentiate CFS from other illnesses and ensure that the patient receives an accurate diagnosis. A correct diagnosis is crucial for developing an effective management plan and improving the patient's quality of life.

WHAT ARE THE MOST EFFECTIVE TREATMENTS FOR CFS?

Treatments for Chronic Fatigue Syndrome focus on managing symptoms and improving quality of life, as there is no one-size-fits-all solution. A multidisciplinary approach is often recommended, involving healthcare providers, physical therapists, and mental health professionals. Key aspects of treatment include managing symptoms through medications, lifestyle adjustments, and therapies that address specific issues such as pain, sleep disturbances, and cognitive difficulties.

Medications may be prescribed to alleviate symptoms such as pain, sleep problems, and depression. Over-the-counter pain relievers or prescription medications may be used for musculoskeletal pain, while sleep aids and cognitive behavioral therapy can help address sleep issues and mood disturbances. Additionally, graded exercise therapy and cognitive behavioral therapy have shown some effectiveness in improving functional outcomes and quality of life for people with CFS.

Lifestyle modifications, including pacing activities, stress management, and dietary adjustments, play a critical role in managing CFS. Patients are encouraged to develop a balanced routine that avoids overexertion and incorporates rest periods. Support from healthcare professionals and peer support groups can also be beneficial in managing the condition and navigating the challenges of daily life.

CAN CFS BE CURED?

Currently, there is no known cure for Chronic Fatigue Syndrome, and management focuses on alleviating symptoms and improving quality of life. Research into the causes and potential cures for CFS is ongoing, but the complexity of the condition means that effective treatments remain elusive. The lack of a definitive cure highlights the importance of ongoing research and individualized treatment plans tailored to each patient's unique symptoms and needs.

Patients with CFS can, however, experience significant improvements in their condition through a combination of symptom management strategies and lifestyle changes.

While a complete cure is not yet available, many individuals find relief through a multidisciplinary approach that includes medical treatment, physical therapy, and psychological support. Success in managing CFS often depends on the patient's ability to adapt to their condition and work collaboratively with their healthcare team.

Continued research into the causes and potential treatments for CFS holds promise for future advancements. In the meantime, managing symptoms effectively and maintaining a supportive healthcare network can help improve the quality of life for those living with CFS.

HOW CAN I FIND SUPPORT FOR MANAGING CFS?

Finding support for managing Chronic Fatigue Syndrome involves accessing resources and networks that provide information, encouragement, and practical assistance. Support can come from healthcare professionals, patient advocacy organizations, and support groups dedicated to CFS. Engaging with these resources can provide valuable information about treatment options, symptom management, and coping strategies.

Healthcare providers can offer personalized treatment plans and refer patients to specialists, such as physical therapists, psychologists, or sleep experts, who can address specific aspects of the condition. Additionally, joining local or online support groups can connect individuals with others facing similar challenges, providing emotional support and practical advice for managing daily life with CFS.

Patient advocacy organizations and online communities can also be valuable sources of information and support. These groups often provide educational resources, updates on research, and forums for sharing experiences and strategies. Engaging with these support systems can help patients navigate the complexities of CFS and find effective ways to manage their symptoms and improve their quality of life.